Ginga And Grow Strong:

I0420459

Improve your Health, Fitness, and Family Life through the art of Brazilian Capoeira

Best Selling Author
CHRIS ROEL

TABLE OF CONTENTS

Legal Notes

Copyright © 2015 CHRIS ROEL

Disclaimer

For Bombada and Reizinho. Thanks for everything!

Ginga and Grow Strong: ®2015

Rei International Publications

*What is Brazilian Capoeira?

Here is a quick note for those who don't know what Brazilian Capoeira is, the other Brazilian Martial Art. Capoeira is a 500 year old martial art created by African slaves in Brazil to practice self-defense under the guise of a dancing game.

It includes a band playing traditional instruments, while a circle of people clap and sing coordinated songs to cheer on the the two practitioners in the middle sparring. This is a very quick generalization of the art for haste's sake.

This book is about the benefits of Capoeira and not the origins or rituals. There is much dispute and variation of these two subjects, but

make no mistake. Capoeira is awesome!

About this Book

This is book is for the average everyday Joe or Jane, considering a martial art or activity to solve one of life's problems, such as weight loss, increasing self-confidence, learning self-defense, muscle and strength building, improving family bonding, seeking to surround yourself with positive influences, or just want to do something cool. Brazilian Capoeira is all of that and more! This book is my story of how I lost 20 pounds, adopted a healthy lifestyle, made life-long successful friends, improved my family life, exposed my wife and son to this magical art form, and embarked on a life improvement journey which would ultimately lead to me becoming not only a published author--but a best selling author.

By the way, did I mention I learned another language, learned how to play Brazilian Percussion, dance Samba, and cook Brazilian cuisine? Well, I did that also, all through Capoeira. We'll get to that in the following pages!

This is not an in-depth technical manual about the intricacies of the secret arts. This is my testimonial that an average overweight guy can take life back beginning with physical self-improvement. There are action requests after each chapter, to explain how you can mirror my results and bonus links to video demonstrations, tutorials, sample diet plan, goal setting sheets, and more.

With these bonuses, you will be introduced to the beautiful art of Brazilian capoeira through music, movement, Culture, language, cuisine. You will begin to know how we live and see the world, and how Capoeira can change your life too.

If you just started training Brazilian Capoeira, this book can guide you inspire you for things to come. I am not the best Capoeirista in the world, but I am very pleased at my level reaching the Graduado cord (black belt), from being a clumsy, out of shape, non-flexible guy. Take a look at this video here and tell me what you think. http://bit.ly/oreivid

If you are my friend, colleague or superior ranking Capoeirista, this book is a good read, and hopefully we can share a laugh at some of my stories about starting this amazing art as just a regular American guy.

You can share this book with your potential students and it should have people knocking at your academy door ready to bring their families in and start training Brazilian Capoeira!

Introduction

Before we begin, let me tell you a little about myself and how Brazilian Capoeira changed my life. Like many people, the first time I saw Capoeira was back in the early 1990's when a C-rate movie popped on cable by the name of "Only the Strong". If you haven't seen this movie, it was a movie produced in the 90's but looked straight out of the 80's. It included cheesy lines, bad acting, and a cliché story line. The movie was about a high school substitute teacher trying to save the worst behavioral students in the school by teaching them martial arts and keeping them off the streets. The main character went on to defeat the local gang leader in hand to hand combat.

There was something different about this version of "Lean of Me", "The Principle", "The Substitute" etc. It featured Brazilian Capoeira--a dancing martial art. Really? I thought this was a Hollywood invention created by a screenwriter with too much time on his hands. The main character danced and flipped while he was fighting. He kicked and swept his opponents while demonstrating amazing acrobatic control of his body.

"Unbelievable", I thought. "For sure it must be fake." It wasn't until years later that while waiting tables in college, I saw a group of

Capoeira students come into the restaurant wearing their white pants, colored rope belts, and t-shirts with a cool Capoeira logo. That's when I knew it was real.

A co-worker of mine said he and his sisters had trained in the art for a couple of months, and that it was awesome, but for some reason he stopped attending classes. Fast forward 5 years later: I was an overweight, college graduate, and new father and looking for a way to lose weight and improve my current non-active lifestyle. My posture was bad and I felt myself slipping away.

I called up the first Capoeira school I found on Google and they never called me back. Two weeks later, I called up the second school I found on Google, and a gentleman called me back within a couple hours and had me set an appointment to come in and try a free class that evening. I never looked back and that was ten years ago from the writing of this book.

Capoeira has given me health (I lost 20 pounds in the first two months), culture (I speak Brazilian Portuguese), a positive lifestyle (my life no longer revolves around bad influences but rather, healthy, active family activities), and so much more we'll get to later in the book.

Whether you looking for a bonding activity for your family, just want to get in shape, or drop a few pounds, looking for a cool martial art and don't like what traditional martial arts offer, or are just curious about this amazing Brazilian cultural sport, this is the book for you. Let's get started!

CHAPTER 1

Chubby Hubby

There I was focused on getting a job right out of college, I was 20 pounds overweight, double chins, potbelly, bad posture, not flexible, I had a newborn son, a wife in college, and an unclear future.

I had never been the chubby guy, but in a matter of 5 years, of a desk job, sedentary lifestyle, too much good food, and a loving fiancé, it happened.

I know that to take back my life, health, and well-being, I had to start with my physical fitness and diet. I tried the ol' weights and running that always worked in the past. I ran 5 miles a day on the treadmill, but it didn't work this time. I had skinny legs and a big belly. "Doh!!!", as Homer Simpson would say.

That's when I decided I needed something high energy. I had played soccer, football and sprinted on the track team in high school, so I knew the value of high-intensity exercise. But there was no way I was gong to join a soccer team, football or track squad. That was just out of the question. I was 26 and already had diminishing daily energy. My infant son would wake up at 5:30 AM, which means we woke up at 5:30 AM. So I knew I had to make a change and take a stand, or I was doomed.

My wife was still in college and not interested in getting in shape, yet. With a newborn, school work, and job waiting tables, it just wasn't on the priority list.

I waited tables at night, took care of my son during the day, meanwhile, searching the net for job opportunities, and sending out my resumé near and far. My mental capacity was starting to diminish along with my posture at 26 years of age. I had to make a plan.

Action Request:

When I was down and out with a family to support, I made the mental decision to change. Whether you're down and out, or just want to improve your current situation, it starts with a plan. Take out a sheet of paper and write out:

3 health goals
3 financial goals
3 personal goals
3 spiritual goals

you would like to accomplish in the next year. You can also click on the link, or enter it into your browser to download my goal planner template

In martial arts, goals are really clear. If you plan to earn your yellow belt, there are listed requirements to meet to achieve it and required action steps that go along with enabling you to do so. Now, list all the possible solutions or actions steps you can think of to achieve your goals. This is a very inspiring exercise. Your mind should be racing with potential answers. Review and work on these daily and we'll come back to this in a later chapter.

http://bit.ly/gingathanks

CHAPTER 2

Ginga

This book is called, "Ginga and Grow Strong" for a reason. The basic movement of which all other attacks, escapes, dodges, and acrobatic movements stem from in Brazilian Capoeira. It is a simple 3-step movement, which if done for more than 20 seconds is pretty demanding in itself.

Below is a diagram of the 3-step movement.

Step one

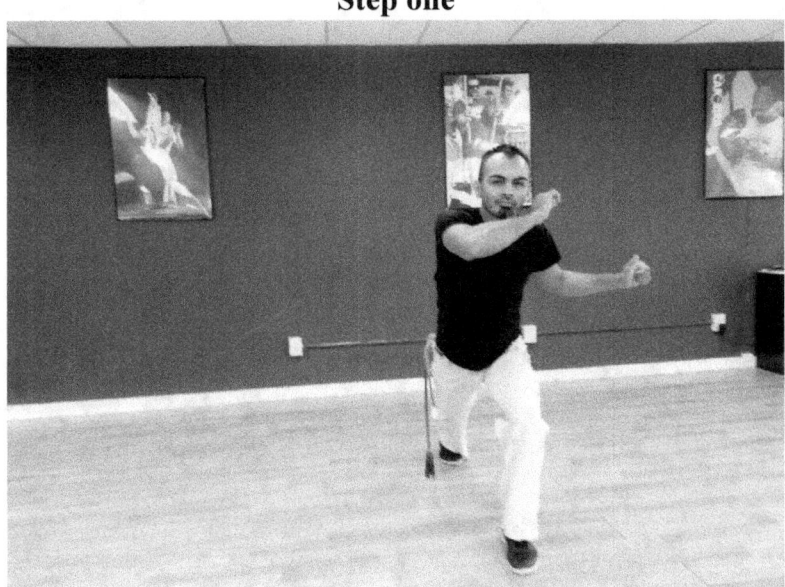

Step Two

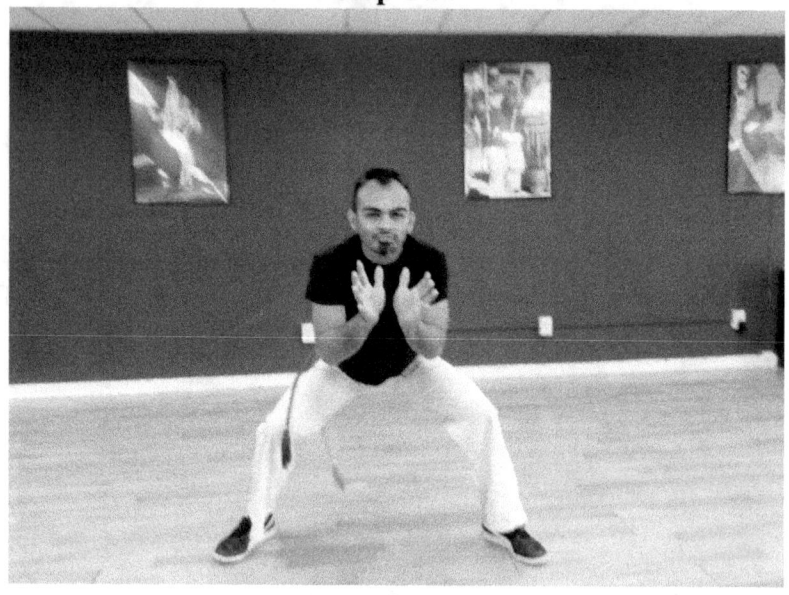

Step Three

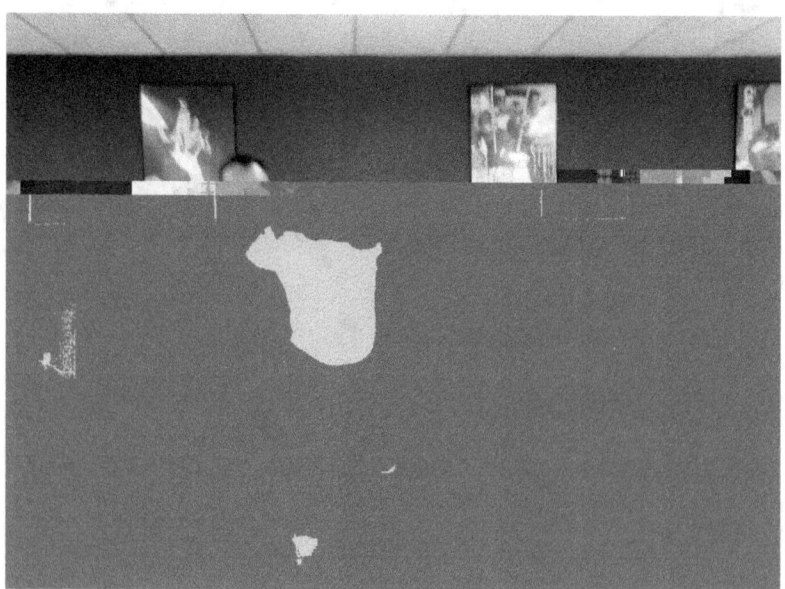

Also click link to see a video demonstration

http://bit.ly/gingathanks

The ginga engages your quads, glutes, hamstrings, calves, arms, core and back. Picture me on my first day of Capoeira class--20 pounds overweight, not flexible, with no rhythm. A very friendly, non-threatening caucasian guy ensured me everything was going to be alright as he coaxed me into the training area.

I just came to watch, but somehow my shoes were off and I was walking into the class that was about to start in seconds. I saw some serious looking dudes in there warming up, but all and a smile on their faces. I felt cautiously safe.

The room smelled of freshly waxed hardwood floor and new paint. There was this smooth Brazilian music playing on the sound system. I was getting pumped up. The vibe was building, but I was still very cautious. Who knew what I was getting myself into in a matter of seconds.

On a quick side note, the only experience I had with the Brazilian culture up to that point was watching the National soccer team dominate in the World Cup on TV. I remember watching the Nike commercial where they dribbled throughout the airport to Samba music. Those guys were pretty cool. Maybe I could be cool too.

Back to me seconds away from my first class, Brazilian music blasting, and students lining up in formation, the instructor stood by me and slowly showed me the 3-step ginga before introducing me to the whole class.

Then it begun, ginga up, down, dodge, cartwheel, lunge, sweep, kick. All the movements were done to the air with minimal partner work. I was drenched in sweat by the first 1/2 hour. This was definitely good exercise and the moves were pretty cool. I was liking this!

The first hour was over and the instructor walked the class over to a cabinet filled with musical instruments. He passed them out to a couple of people and had us others clap along. "We were really going to learn the Brazilian music", I thought to myself.

He taught a song in Portuguese to the class. Nothing hard, just one or two sentences long. "We were really learning music in Portuguese", I thought again. Right after that, we began to circle up and they began playing those instruments again while students took turns sparring each other in the middle two at a time.

They pushed me in and although I was very nervous, I can say I enjoyed it. That was 10 years ago and I've been ginga-ing ever since.

There was something about the playfulness of the art, the happy, positive, people, the culture, music, language, a healthy lifestyle, everything altogether that helped me improve my health, fitness, outlook on life, circle of friends, family relations, and so much more.

It all started with the "Ginga"...

Action Request:

Click the link or post in your browser and try the following easy exercises with Ginga and a few dodges.

http://bit.ly/gingathanks

Ginga 5x each side

esquiva

esquiva lateral

quebrada

Also, if you haven't already done so, weigh yourself (you don't have to tell anyone) and write it down. Take your waist size and write it down. If you're considering Capoeira as a weight loss solution, then we have to track where we start at so we can see improvement.

CHAPTER 3

Music and Brazilian Portuguese

Well, like I said before, I signed up and never looked back. I dropped 20 pounds in 2 months. One of the reasons I had such amazing results was because I enjoyed the class so much. That was because of the music and language aspect. Yeah, the moves were cool, and yes the exercises, although self-paced, were pretty demanding. The Music gave all of that purpose.

For those of you all who don't know, the Capoeira circle in which two students spar, called a roda (pronounced ho-dah), is controlled by the music, instruments, and lyrics of the bateria (band). They dictate whether the sparring session will be fast or slow, playful or more combat orientated.

This book isn't about the ancient rituals of the Capoeira circle, or else I could go on and on, but let me explain that the music is an essential element of it. Without the music, it would be karate, or gymnastics, or something else not capoeira.

Here are a few names of Capoeira Masters and artists you can Google or search on Youtube that will definitely please your ear:

Mestre Accordeon

Mestre Suassuna

Carolina Soares

Axé Capoeira (Mestre Barrão)

Capoeira builds this lifestyle of training movements and strikes, cultural exploration, language learning, and healthy diet and lifestyle. By the end of the first year, I spoke and understood a lot of Portuguese just through music learning in Capoeira alone. My instructor was a white guy who went to BYU for crying out loud. This stuff really works!

Action Request:

Do a Youtube music search on the artists mentioned above. There are several playlists and videos you can enjoy, but I recommend Mestre Accordeon, first. His music is more mainstream sounding and easy on non-Brazilian ears for their first time.

Also, click http://bit.ly/gingathanks or paste in your browser for your bonus crash course on Brazilian Portuguese so you can enjoy the music better. Don't worry it won't be too complicated or time-consuming. Usually in Capoeira class one or two songs are taught per week so that it allows time for it to sink in. Enjoy a new song taught each chapter from now on. Thanks and see you in the next chapter.

CHAPTER 4

Life Improvement...Go!

Two months later I was 20 pounds lighter, clear headed, happy and inspired in life. I had secured a job at a lab using my Science degree and was climbing life's ladder. I was training Capoeira only twice a week and lifting weights and running twice a week. It was a good balance and I was the fittest I had ever been in my life.

Now remember, I played high school football and in Texas that means hard core training weights, cardio, and torture. I may had been buffer and bulkier in high school, but it felt like superficial muscles. From Capoeira, I was strong from the core out plus with self-defense and martial arts aspects, I was even more self-confident and, even better, I was a more respectful human being.

Learning honor, loyalty, self-control really helped enlighten me.

I lifted weights because I wanted to remain active on my non-Capoeira days and I was really and truly inspired to get better. I would do a Capoeira warm-up, stretch, hit the treadmill, then the weights.

You can get results with the regimen I'm going to give you to change your life for the better. Also diet is super important which I'll get to in a later chapter. You just can't eat like a pig and exercise. This isn't a get slim quick scam or a fad diet. It is an amazing change in lifestyle that's fun and has multiple benefits and is extremely life enrichening.

I mentioned that I lost 20 pounds in the first 2 months, but guess what? I lost an additional 10 pounds. When I started doing aerial acrobatics! It was all that body and core muscle constriction while in the air.

I don't expect everyone to flip and fly in the air, but I wanted to note the potential for results with this art. My self-confidence was fly flying. I felt great. I loved my fiancé and son. I was working towards goals, and I was more respectful, disciplined and cultured human being. I'm going to recommend to you that you think about your personal values. To make an external change, you must first change internally. The way you live your life must be congruent with your internal values. We have a saying in martial arts:

"Dogs share the same fleas"

This means that if you hang out with people who drink, do drugs, stay out all night, overeat, and are unfaithful in their personal relationships, you too will sooner or later share the same behavior as them.

Invest in yourself and in your family. Improve your values and shun those bad influences who may be your good friends or family members. I took a stand and parted from my college buddies who just worked and drank their paychecks at the bar, staying out all night chasing women that made them wake up late barely in time to take a shower and race to work.

My life was improving, as will yours, when I dedicated myself to improving myself personally--health and fitness, loyalty to my family and positive lifestyle, surrounding myself with positive like-minded goal orientated people, and finally spiritual improvement.

Whether you're Catholic, Protestant, Muslim, Jewish, Buddhist, or Atheist, I recommend you exercise your spiritual muscles also. I'm not going to rant, but at least some meditation should be practiced to reflect on your improvement and gratitude towards all the great things in your life we will touch on this in a later chapter.

For now, let's get you back to improving your life.

Action Request:

Click on the link to see the group of Capoeira exercises. This is slightly more vigorous, but you are ready. http:// bit.ly/gingathanks

Also included is the song of the chapter in Brazilian Portuguese.

Write on a piece of paper your current values. For example, honest, loyal, hardworking, self-disciplined, religious, health conscious, etc. and contemplate daily how your actions are or are not congruent with them. Is it time for a change?

CHAPTER 5

Esquiva

As you have seen already, Capoeira uses a lot of dodging rather than blocking. That's what makes this art so fluid and smooth, and one great core workout.

This goes along with the philosophy of Capoeira. For example, a lot of new students what should they do if they were caught in a dark alley in the middle of the night and an attacker approaches. We say to this, "What are you doing in a dark alley in the middle of the night in the first place?" That's exactly where attackers hang out.

Avoid the situation. Avoid the attack. Don't be there when the strike or kick is. That's the way you should live your life. Don't be there for the bad influences, bad habits, and bad lifestyles.

We will now proceed with a kicking and dodging exercise as follows. Make sure you know the names of the following dodges and kicks or you can review them on the previous link given.

Esquiva Left: left-hand flat on the ground, right leg straight back, left hand protecting the face, and left leg bent and solid on the ground.

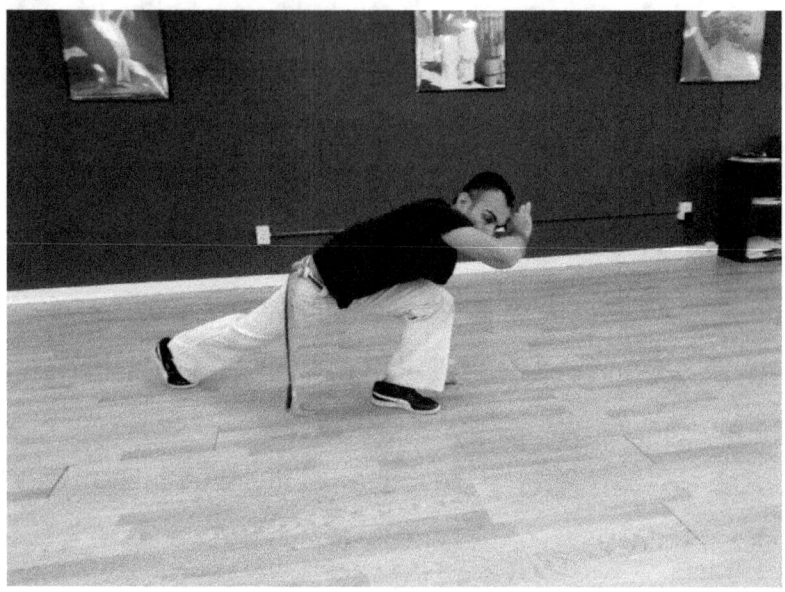

Esquiva Right: right-hand flat on the ground, left leg straight back, right hand protecting the face, and right leg bent and solid on the ground.

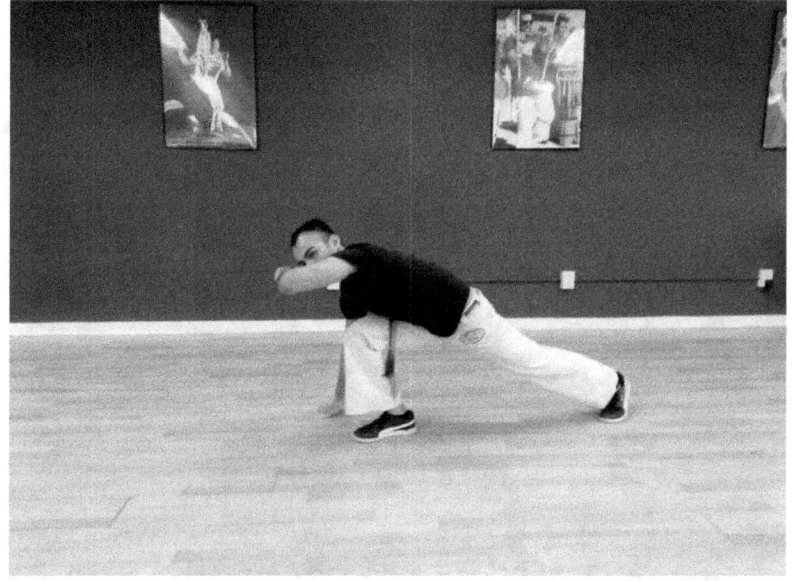

Esquiva Lateral Left

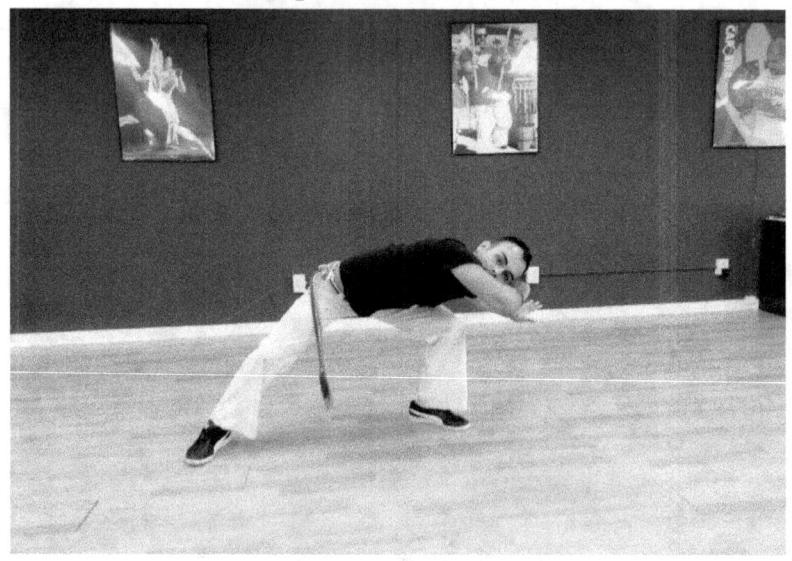

Esquiva Lateral Right

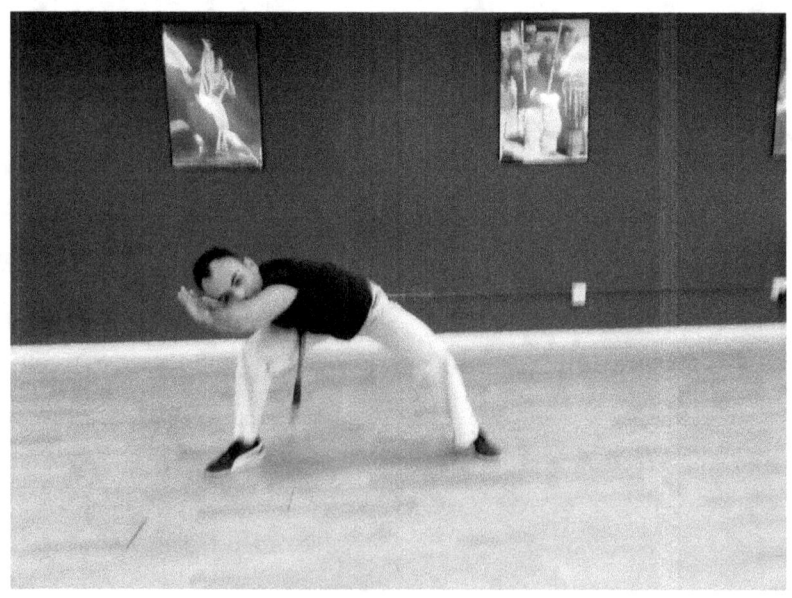

Quebrada Left: Perpendicular to opponent, front hand protecting, back hand back, posture low, straight back, bent leg

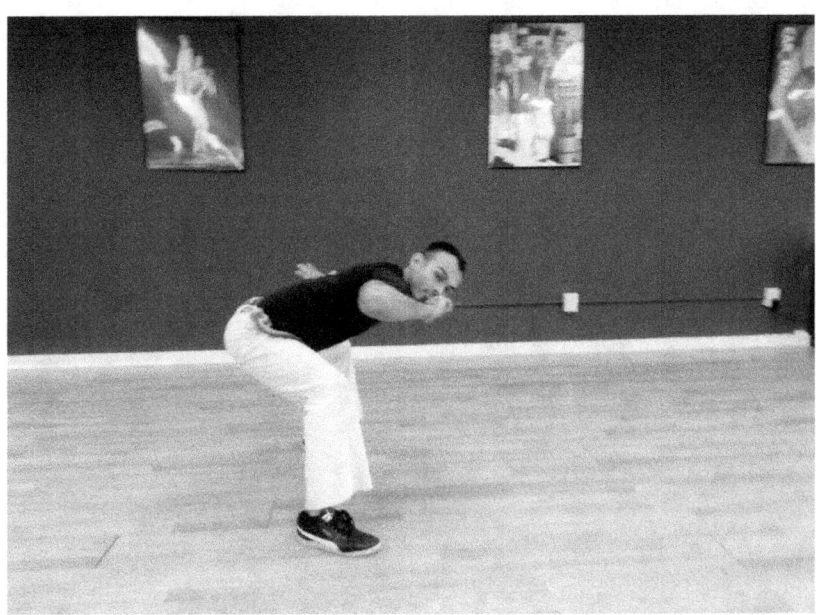

Quebrada Right: Perpendicular to opponent, front hand protecting, back hand back, posture low, straight back, bent legs

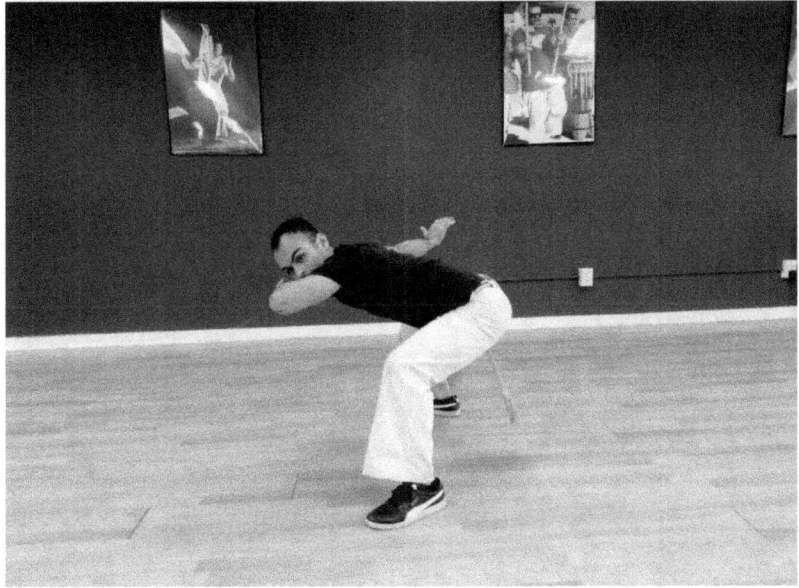

Ginga-esquiva, step up, martelo (both sides 5x each)

Ginga -esquiva lateral, meia lua de frente (both sides 5x each)
Ginga-quebrada, benção

Action Request:

Do the exercises listed above. You can click the link http://bit.ly/ gingathanks or paste in your browser for a demonstration.

Make a list of bad influences in your life you need to esquiva (dodge) and reflect on it.

CHAPTER 6

The Family that Kicks Together Sticks Together

As I was coming up the ranks at my Capoeira academy, I didn't notice how many happy families training together in class. I was too involved in my own fun training. In hindsight, however, it is all clear now.

They would kick and dodge with each other, do a cartwheel, laugh and carry on. It was amazing. It only occurred to me when my son became old enough to start training. He turned 4 years old and started attending Capoeira classes. It was the best thing that happened, that even overshadowed my own awesome experience.

He loved the music, the acrobatics, the martial arts, the playful game aspect of it. Most martial arts can be intimidating for a child, but Capoeira is taught as a game. It totally disarms any worries that a child or adult might have. Most everyone is respectful and not malicious. They want to help beginners get better without trying to hurt them.

Low contact and more dodging rather than hard blocking make it very attractive to people trying to avoid injury. Sure enough, in time, confidence builds, the student is desensitized to takedowns and contact at their own pace. They build acrobatic core strength, body control, rhythm, flexibility, compassion and so much more.

My son started to excel and draw attention from the extended family. It was only a matter of time, that my wife signed up, too. We all started training together, bonding, laughing and playing with each other.

I didn't need to punch my wife in the face, or choke her out like other martial arts training might involve, but rather play and paw at her and my son. They would dodge out of the way safely and escape with a cartwheel. We share a smile and laugh.

We got in the best shape of our lives and adopted super healthy lifestyles. We practiced music together, Portuguese, cartwheels and bridges, healthy dieting, and even supplemental weight training.

My son, as any kid exposed to an activity young, has excelled in this art. He flips, bends sings, dances, and grows strong! It has created an awesome dynamic in our family. We sweat, train play, laugh, flip, sing, pray, and grow strong together. I'm not the first family to enjoy this. There are husbands, wives, and kids practicing capoeira all over the world. They enjoy the same benefits I have and some more! My mentors before me and my students currently are living the Capoeira lifestyle! We travel all over the country to Capoeira events, having a great time.   Through Capoeira, our traveling turns into mini-vacations and our vacations into mini-Capoeira explorations.

It's true, "The Family that kicks together, Sticks together".

Action Request:

Click the next lesson http://bit.ly/gingathanks or paste in your browser.

Feel your life getting better and your body getting stronger.

-Bridge push ups and rotations

-Macacos

-Aus

-Roles

-Kicks into each

CHAPTER 7

Diet

It is true that there is no magic button for weight loss and health, but the same old combination of diet and exercise. You must change your lifestyle to one that's congruent with your values, so you may any long lasting results.

It even came out of my own mouth at the time I was living an unhealthy lifestyle, "I want to eat what I want! There's no way I'm giving up cheeseburgers and frito pies!"

Then I changed my values. I valued my own health more than temporary joy from fat foods. Whatever healthy food and drink I began consuming from that point on, my body perceived it as good tasting. I enjoyed non-sugared beverages like water, unsweet tea, and coffee with no sweetener.

No sodas or carbonated sugar drinks. They have no nutritional value. Just water (lots of it), juices, and milk (optional). Lay off the alcohol. It'll help you drop weight and give you a clear mind to focus on achieving your goals.

Take supplemental vitamins. No need to get fancy, just the one-a-day kind from the grocery store, maybe some fish oil if you pushing 30 years of age.

I recommend a whey protein shake either as an after training meal(at night) or a breakfast snack. If you train at night, you'll need some carbs for energy an hour before class. Grilled chicken and rice, or sweet potatoes will do nicely.

Throw out everything fried. Sorry, no french fries, onion rings, fried chicken, etc. Eat lean meats like grilled fish, chicken, turkey. Fruits, green vegetables. This will get you started. This is how I lost 20 pounds in the first two months and felt great! I had increasing energy each day to achieve my goals.

Now I know it seems that we don't have time to cook, or prepare meals, or seek out healthy options. Let me give you a great tip if you can't avoid the fast food restaurants. During my first years of training capoeira, I worked at Chili's waiting tables and I could not avoid eating fast food either quickly before or after a long shift. I got creative. Most fast food restaurants have a fish sandwich--get that and throw out the greasy bread. Most places have grilled chicken sandwich--do the same with that one. Also, nowadays most places have a mixed fruit cup or parfait. Don't get all of the sugar toppings. Be smart and stay disciplined. Remember your body is a machine. You want it to burn clean fuel. Think longevity--30 years of burgers and fries or 30 years of clean meat and veggies? Don't forget--water, water, water! Flush and repeat.

Action Request:

Click the link to download a sample diet plan or post it in your browser. http://bit.ly/gingathanks

We want you to be very conscious on what you put in your body, whether you're trying to lose weight, build muscle or just live healthier. Being introduced to the Brazilian culture, I was pleasantly pleased to find out how much fresh fruit the Brazilians and South Americans eat. Pineapples, passion fruit, kiwis, açai, bananas, and more.

Try to cut out bad foods mentioned before and add at least three good foods and supplements from the chapter this week.

CHAPTER 8

Character Development for Kids and Adults

Probably the number one reason why Brazilian Capoeira causes most students to be successful in their personal life is the character development. I will list and describe briefly a few traits learned through going through a Brazilian Capoeira program.

Focus-focus when the instructor is teaching, when your muscles are aching, when your drenched in sweat when the music is blaring. This translates to focus in the classroom, when distractions are high and when it's time to perform. It translates to focus on the job when the boss is mad, and assignment is due, when a deadline approaching when your productivity and commission depend on it.

Discipline- to do what you have to do when you have to do it, whether you feel like it or not. Discipline to finish your drills when you're tired when you feel lazy, or when you're sad. This translates to finishing assignments and homework instead of TV or video games, or cell phones and calling friends.

It translates to going to Capoeira class when friends are going to the bar for happy hour when friends are going out to eat or the movies. It translates to saving your money and investing it, instead of overspending. Budgeting when you really want to go on a shopping spree.

Respect-respect for your instructor, for your Mestre, your superior ranking classmates. Respect for your teachers and adults, and authority. Respect for the law and law officials and people's property. Respect for your boss, colleagues, family, and clients. Respect for your body and others' bodies. Respect for you mind.

Loyalty-loyalty to your Capoeira group, Mestre, and instructor. This translates to loyalty your friends, spouse or future spouse. Loyalty to your future family and children. Loyalty to your religion and God.

These character traits are, I believe, the driving factors for producing positive upbeat, goal driven, successful people with great family lives.

Action Request:
Try to push yourself on the following Capoeira training. Make yourself finish despite the vigor. Push toward achieving one of your written down goals from the earlier chapter.

http://bit.ly/gingathanks

CHAPTER 9

Choosing the Right Capoeira School

So you have decided to train Capoeira? Well, it's pretty awesome with several life benefits, but what will you look for in a Capoeira dojo? Let's talk about some things to consider. There are some amazing Capoeira masters out there who can teach you amazing things and that keep things pretty traditional to the way they do it in Brazil. There are teachers out there who aren't masters but are black belts (graduados/instrutores/monitores). And then there are student teachers--students who have or haven't the permission from their master to teach this awesome art.

Capoeira is pretty scarce compared to karate or BJJ, but it has grown drastically in the last 10 years. Do you want a family friendly group? Then make sure the dojo is congruent with your family values. Some have amazing adult programs but aren't suitable for children.

There are a few different styles Brazilian Capoeira: Angola, Contemporenea, and Regional. Although Angola can be fast, it is usually classified as the slow style of Capoeira. It is low to the ground and very ceremonial.

Contemporenea groups are the most popular. They are the faster upright and more acrobatic type of capoeira. It is an evolution of the Regional style in modern day times.

Regional groups play what is considered to be the traditional type of Capoeira created by Mestre Bimba.

There are groups that teach all styles and some just stick to one style. As a beginner, go and visit a couple academy's to see if it fits what you're looking for. If choices are limited in your city, well, you gotta do what you gotta do. Most groups will still have everything your looking for and more.

Expect to what at least 6 months to a year for your first belt, but you may be able to slip in at the right time in some groups and earn your first belt in a couple months. Belts are given at events called Batizados, or baptisms. Some groups don't give belts, you just train until they say you're an instructor or professor.

Action Request:
Click the link http://bit.ly/gingathanks or post in your browser to see a school locator. You can find several in your area all over the world. Go visit one and try a class!

CHAPTER 10

Summary

I hope this book has inspired you to make a positive change in your life, and to get you to try a Capoeira class in your area. Like I said previously, it can solve many of life's problems. This beautiful flamboyant art is not only for the outgoing and athletic. It is for everyday Joes and Janes, like me and you.

It took me from an uncoordinated out of shape dad to a flexible, agile, acrobatic martial artist, linguist, and musician. I am very happy with what Capoeira has given me, but I'm not even a top level Capoeira. There are people who have dedicated themselves to mastering this beautiful art, physically and culturally. That could be you.

My happiness comes from that it improved my personal life, not just my physical. I have made great life-long friends and mentors. I have mentored hundreds in the right direction, and I can say that is my biggest accomplishment. I have improved my family's and my lives so much and can give back to the community.

It helped me pursue a lifelong dream of becoming a published author. I went on to start my own business and do what I love, living a healthy lifestyle. Without it, I may have just floundered at my teaching job for 20 years and collect my pension. With the support of my Capoeira community I became a best selling author with my book on Capoeira for Brazilian Jiu-Jitsu. Owning and running a business is tough and it's not for everyone but I'm glad I embarked on this journey.

You could be the next happy family training Capoeira and feeling the best in your life. You can be the next cool mom that all the other moms are talking about while at their plane ol' Zumba class. You can be the next mentor inspiring others to train Capoeira and be the best they can be, in and outside the dojo, pursuing your dreams.

Thanks again and get out there and Ginga!

BONUS CHAPTER

As I was finishing writing this book, I noticed I didn't pay enough respect at how amazing Capoeira is for kids. This book was aimed at the adult who wants to overcome their current situation and include their family, but Brazilian Capoeira is really beneficial for kids.

There is so much more activity in it compared to a regular traditional martial arts program of just kicking and punching. The cool movements, acrobatics, music and languages skills really blast a kid's confidence. A confident kid is usually a bully repellent kid. This is a whole other book to itself that I can go on and on about. The same things that I mentioned for the adults and families.

At the Capoeira school that I own, we really concentrate on developing kids. These kids are flipping and flying, singing in Portuguese, playing the instruments, dancing Samba, and everything else we have to offer.

If you are considering Capoeira for your child, then do it. Sign him/her up and then try Capoeira yourself and take your spouse. It really is something you can practice safely with your whole family. We've had several families come through our studio and LOVE it!

I hope this book has been helpful to you and help you make a decision. I hope the tutorial videos, printouts, demonstrations, and sample Portuguese lessons have really added value to this book. I wanted to slam back this book with so much extra value that it would really do justice of our beautiful art.

If you are a single guy/gal with no kids, even better. You can concentrate all your efforts to getting better in this addictive art. Do not, however, use the dojo for a meat market. Many people have met through Capoeira and have dated and gotten married. It is truly something special to witness.

Girls don't want to get hit on when they're trying to work out and other mothers don't want girls flaunting their stuff in a family environment if they have children training there. Just be respectful and smart. If you're looking for a buff Capoeira stud, you may be training for the wrong reasons, even though there may be plenty of hard bodies.

If you're looking for a ripped girlfriend, you're probably going to get dropped or blasted by the instructor. You don't want to get on the bad side of a martial arts instructor, so focus on yourself and you'll get more out of it.

I tried to give you a little taste of the amazing experience you will have when you go to a real Brazilian Capoeira studio. Like I mentioned earlier in the book, it will be even more awesome in person. This is not a substitution for joining a school. I really recommend that after reading this book, you use our link to a school locator in your area, or do an internet search. Well, good luck God bless.

<u>Thanks for Reading</u>

I hope this book has inspired you to find a Capoeira dojo near you and try a class! If you can't find anything near you , a good academy is worth a drive. We've had students in our group drive an hour and a half both ways to train. If that's not feasible for your situations. Check out some of my other products coming soon at

www.gingaandgrowstrong.com

Other Works by Best Selling Author Chris Roel

"Ginga and Roll Strong: 10 Capoeira Exercises to Improve Your BJJ"

"O Rei's Capoeira Ground Game System: From Beginner to Intermediate Level"

Coming Soon

"The 7 Habits of Highly Successful Capoeira Students: Take your Capoeira and Life to the Next level"

"Eat and Ginga Strong: Brazilian Capoeira Diet for Health, Weight Loss, and Longevity"

"Ginga and Build Confidence: Deflect Bullies with Brazilian Capoeira Techniques, Philosophy, and Lifestyle"

If you are in the Corpus Christi, Texas area, then you owe it to yourself to come visit our amazing academy where we have been transforming lives big and small. Visit www.capcorpus.com. Your life could be the next one that Capoeira changes for the better!

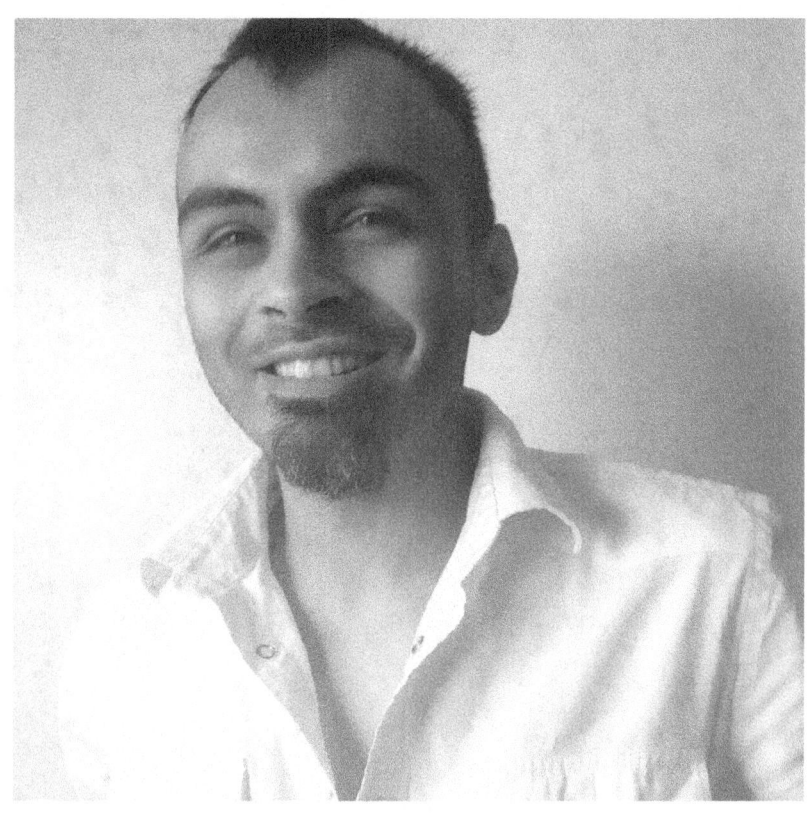

About the Author

Chris Roel started training Brazilian Capoeira in San Antonio TX, with CapuraGinga Capoeira under Professor Advogado, in 2006. He has trained all over the United States with various masters of Capoeira. He has taught classes and workshops and run multiple Capoeira schools in Texas. He currently owns and operates a Brazilian Capoeira school in Corpus Christi TX with his wife and son. He helps his students reach their potential inside and outside of the dojo through the character development techniques of Capoeira. He is known as O Rei in the Capoeira community.